CANCER AND NATURAL DIETS AND NUTRITION

By David Schultz

Contents

CHAPTER 1. FUNDAMENTAL FACTS OF CANCER 6

CHAPTER 2. THE END OF COMMON DISEASES 8

CHAPTER 3. WHAT IS CANCER 13

CHAPTER 4. HOW CANCER DIAGNOSED 21

CHAPTER 5. NATURAL REMEDY FOR CANCER 24

CHAPTER 6. CARE GIVING FOR YOUR LOVED ONE 39

CHAPTER 7. 7 KEY RISK FACTORS FOR CANCERS YOU MUST KNOW 50

CHAPTER 8. THE CANCER SIGNS 53

CHAPTER 9. FIVE ALL-STAR FOODS TO HELP PREVENT CANCER 58

Copyright 2016 by Dr. David Shultz - All rights reserved.

This document is geared towards providing exact and reliable information in regards to the topic and issue covered. The publication is sold with the idea that the publisher is not required to render accounting, officially permitted, or otherwise, qualified services. If advice is necessary, legal or professional, a practiced individual in the profession should be ordered.

- From a Declaration of Principles which was accepted and approved equally by a Committee of the American Bar Association and a Committee of Publishers and Associations.

In no way is it legal to reproduce, duplicate, or transmit any part of this document in either electronic means or in printed format. Recording of this publication is strictly prohibited and any storage of this document is not allowed unless with written permission from the publisher. All rights reserved.

The information provided herein is stated to be truthful and consistent, in that any liability, in terms of inattention or otherwise, by any usage or abuse of any policies, processes, or directions contained within is the solitary and utter responsibility of the recipient reader. Under no circumstances will any legal responsibility or blame be held against the publisher for any reparation, damages, or monetary loss due to the information herein, either directly or indirectly.

Respective authors own all copyrights not held by the publisher.

The information herein is offered for informational purposes solely, and is universal as so. The presentation of the information is without contract or any type of guarantee assurance.

The trademarks that are used are without any consent, and the publication of the trademark is without permission or backing by the trademark owner. All trademarks and brands within this book are for clarifying purposes only and are the owned by the owners themselves, not affiliated with this document.

Disclaimer

Due to the laws and rules regarding health and wellness, the medical establishment has made it very difficult for anyone to even mention the word "cure" next to a disease or illness. Even though what you are about to read has been studied for decades, proven and researched as fact by medical doctors, scientists, researchers, dieticians, nutritionists, and may just as well "cure" you and restore your full health, by law we are not allowed to do so or say so. Thus, the law requires us to state the following:

This book is not in any way offered as prescription, diagnosis nor treatment for any disease, illness, infirmity or physical condition. Any form of self-treatment or alternative health program necessarily must involve an individual's acceptance of some risk, and no one should assume otherwise. Persons needing medical care should obtain it from a physician. Consult your doctor or health practitioner before making any health decision.

All material in this book is provided for your information only and may not be construed as medical advice or instruction. No action or inaction should be taken based solely on the contents of this information; instead, readers should consult appropriate health professionals on any matter relating to their health and well-being.

The information and opinions expressed here are believed to be accurate, based on the best judgment available to the authors; and readers who fail to consult with appropriate health authorities assume the risk of any injuries. No warranty or guarantee of a cure is expressed or implied with any information in this book. In no event shall the author, 7 Steps to Health, The ICTM, its employees or associates be liable to any person or individual for any loss or damage whatsoever which may arise from the use of the information in this book. To put it simply before doing anything, make sure to consult your doctor. Contact the author with any questions or suggestions at drdsr@dr.com

NOTES TO THE READER

While the writers of this book have endeavored sensible endeavors to guarantee the exactness and timeliness of the data contained in this book, the writer and distributer expect no risk concerning misfortune or harm brought on, or charged to be created, by any dependence on any data contained thus and repudiate all guarantees, communicated or inferred, with regards to the precision or dependability of said data. This production is intended to give exact and legitimate data with respect to the topic secured.

INTRODUCTION

Though we have all heard the term "Cancer" through many sources, the exact facts and details of the disease are not very widely known. Cancer is one of the world's deadliest diseases and is a completely curable if detected at an early stage. It is, therefore, a must to possess awareness about it and this eBook is a consolidation of the facts and details related to this disease.

CHAPTER 1. FUNDAMENTAL FACTS OF CANCER

To get sick, to be confined in the hospital, to pay for hospitals bills, to take medications for the rest of the life are among man's most hated occurrences. This is the reality of our life. We can never escape sickness especially when a certain disease runs in the family's blood. If you have a hereditary predisposition of a certain type of disease, there is a great possibility that you can pass it to your future children and to the next generations. If it runs in the blood, you can never lose your track from it.

Cancer, as we all know, is a hereditary disease that is very life threatening. Up to this point, there is still no cure for the disease. But let us not lose hope since the disease can still be managed through a couple of therapies and of course, faith. Nothing is lost if you just believe in the power of faith and with the ability of the medications and therapies to manage the type of cancer an individual has.

It is shocking to know that cancer strikes at any age, but it does strike more frequently in the later years. Even the little ones cannot escape the disease and it is just sad to know that many little children have spared their life after suffering from a certain type of cancer. Many factors are believed to have contributed to the development of cancer. These cancer factors include frictional and chemical irritations like smoking and irritations of the skin and mouth. Exposure to the direct heat of the sun X-rays or any other radioactive elements can also contribute to the development of cancer.

The most common body organs that are affected by cancer are the lungs, pancreas, kidney, bladder, skin, and uterus, breast for women and prostate for men. When the client has lung cancer, the cancer cells does not only metastasize in the lungs but it will metastasize to other vital organs if not treated promptly.

Early detection and prompt treatment are considered the best protection against cancer. When you are diagnosed as having a certain type of cancer, you feel so shocked that it feels like you were hit by zap stun gun. You feel so shocked that you wished for the physician to take back what he said. All you have to do is to just accept the hurtful fact and face the disease bravely.

But what will be your basis for consulting the physician? There are these warning signs of cancer that will determine if the individual may or may do not have cancer. These warning signs include unusual bleeding or discharges, a lump or thickening in the breast or any part of the body, a sore that does not seem to heal unexplainable weight loss, frequent headaches, hoarseness of voice or a cough and change in the bowel or bladder habits. If you have experienced any of these warning signs, immediately consult the physician for immediate action and treatment.

Patients with cancer undergo several types of therapy depending on the severity of the disease. Surgery may do as well. Chemotherapy and radiation therapy are the most common treatments for cancer. When you have undergone several courses of therapies, your body gets too tired that it seems you were hit by a stunning master a couple of times. Still, you need to believe and constantly pray for a miracle. Anything is possible just as long as you have a strong faith and is very determined to survive cancer.

CHAPTER 2. THE END OF COMMON DISEASES

This photo shows the most recent accessible insights from the World Health Organization with respect to the primary driver of death in Europe, the United States, and other industrialized nations toward the finish of the twentieth century. Consistently 12 million individuals overall bite the dust of the consequences of atherosclerosis, heart areas of dead tissue, and strokes. These are by a long shot the most widely recognized reasons for the death of our time. Cell Medicine has effectively found a response to this pandemic: atherosclerosis and its outcomes, heart dead tissue and stroke are early types of scurvy. In light of this learning, coronary illness will be decreased to a small amount of the present figures throughout the following decades.

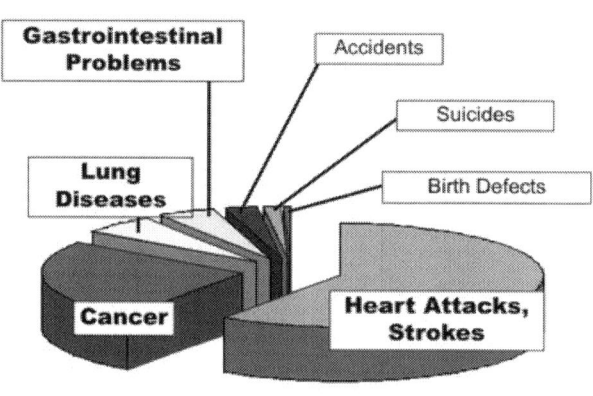

Eight out of ten people die of coronary heart disease or cancer

The second-biggest regular disease is cancer malignant tumors. Coronary illness and tumor together are in charge of more than 80% of all deaths in industrialized nations. Frequencies of disease continue expanding on a worldwide scale. There is just a single conceivable clarification for this: ordinary drug does not know the reasons for growth nor how this sickness spreads. In light of this, there is no viable tumor treatment accessible and the ailment can continue developing a global scale.

The most well-known diseases and causes of death in developing nations are irresistible ailments, including the AIDS scourge. These genuinely irresistible infections can just keep spreading the way they do in light of the fact that the information of cell wellbeing has been not productively utilized. This book will likewise give the answer for the control of these infections.

Common Diseases and Causes of Death

The Fundamental Question of Cellular Health: Where Does the Problem Originate in a Cell?

Fundamentally, the root of the disease can be considered from two cell perspectives: the absence of organic fuel required by the cell's energy plants, the mitochondria, or a disappointment in the capacity of the core, the metabolic control focus of the cell.

Absence of natural fuel in the power plants of the cell (mitochondria)

Coronary heart disease, for example, is primarily brought about by an inadequate supply to the cell of organic fuel as vitamins and other cell elements. These supplements are required for the change of sustenance into cell vitality, which is utilized by the cell in numerous metabolic responses. Another illustration is heart disappointment, which is brought about by an absence of bio-fuel in the cells of the heart muscle. With low vitality creation, the pumping capacity of the heart muscle gets to be distinctly debilitated, bringing about shortness of breath and the aggregation of liquids in the body. For the most part, the supply of vitamins and other bio-vitality fuel will revise the disabled pumping capacity of the heart muscle.

Diseases caused on by an issue in the cell's metabolic program

The second biggest reason for diseases, in general, is a mistake in the metabolic programming of the cell's control focus, the core. Like a computer virus that will disrupt a computer's ordinary capacities, cells can fall under the control of a malady program. Essential sicknesses in this gathering are irresistible maladies, (for example, infection diseases) and growth. This defective programming will prompt to an illness just when two preconditions have been met:

Programming mistake causes uncontrolled "cell duplication," and in the meantime,

Programming mistake causes a "disturbance of the association of the encompassing connective tissue," which empowers the sick cells to spread.

The mechanisms that encourage the spread of these forceful sicknesses and the conceivable outcomes of backing off or ceasing their advance will be talked about later in detail.

Diseases Originate Inside the Cells

Most common cause of disease:
Lack of Biological Fuel in the Cell Power Plant

A lack of bio-energy carriers (vitamins, minerals, trace elements) in the powerplants of the cell (mitochondria)

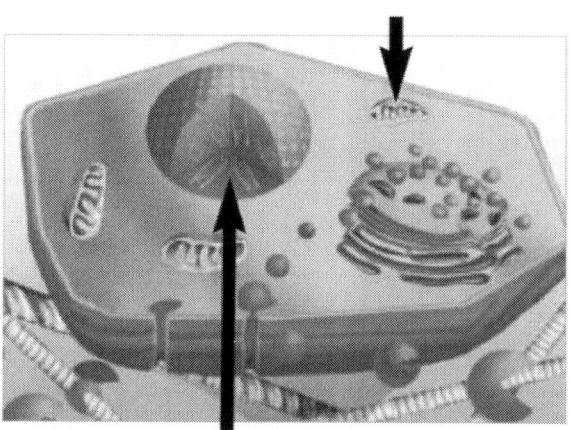

Second most common cause of disease:
Reprogramming of the cell's control system

How Cells Move Through the Body

In the event that we need to see how disease spreads in the body, we need to investigate the way cells travel through the body. This is anything but difficult to clarify on account of red and white platelets: these cells are quite recently conveyed along in the circulatory system. Be that as it may, it is harder to envision how cells forming different organs can travel through a body's solid connective tissue. This happens each second inside our bodies.

Keeping in mind the end goal to travel through the connective tissue, any cell must be able to do briefly dissolving the encompassing tissue the collagen and versatile filaments - so it can advance through. For this reason, the cells utilize catalysts that can incidentally process and debilitate the connective strands encompassing them. All compounds are proteins, which are created by the cells themselves and after that emitted. So as to end up distinctly dynamic, numerous chemicals tie to other particular particles, for example, follow components, which change their biochemical structure and prompt their action. Cell movement through thick tissue requires that the cell emits compounds that can disintegrate the encompassing collagen. This is the reason these protein atoms are known as collagen-processing catalysts.

What's more, the cell regularly needs to secrete activators the atoms that can vitalize lethargic catalysts situated outside the cell, empowering them to process and extricate up the encompassing collagen particles.

Cell Movements through Body Tissue

Collagen-Dissolving Cell Systems

Most cells of the body are equipped for delivering chemicals that can "eat" their way through connective tissue. In solid individuals this happens in certain, naturally characterized physiological stages. In an infection, this happens when cells and cell frameworks get to be reinvented. Malignancy cells, for example, utilize these "natural weapons" to duplicate inside an organ and after that spread through the whole body (metastasis). Infections and different microorganisms additionally utilize this collagen-dissolving "weapon" to spread a contamination to different parts of the body.

A — Cell nucleus initiates the production of enzymes that dissolve collagen
- Production of these enzymes in the cell
- Secretion of enzymes into the surrounding tissue
- Enzyme molecules making their way through collagen fibers of the tissue

B —
- Tissue around the cell is *temporarily dissolved*
- Cell can move through body tissue

How is it conceivable that a solitary disease system - the decimation of collagen by protein-processing catalysts is of such remarkable esteem that it assumes an imperative part in all genuine infections? The body itself utilizes a similar system in a sound individual for its typical capacities, in different metabolic pathways or to rebuild certain organs. For example, enzymatic debasement of the connective tissue is vital in the capacity of the body's safe framework, amid development, furthermore in the rebuilding of the regenerative organs amid the month to month female cycle and in pregnancy.

Nonetheless, our bodies are completely helpless when the instrument that it ordinarily utilizes gets to be distinctly actuated and mishandled, for example, by attacking microorganisms. When the infection or growth cell is equipped for beating the body with its own particular collagen-dissolving weapons, the sickness begins spreading aggressively.

To clarify this essential rule that recognizes our health from disease, we will take a gander at how the body utilizes this collagen-dissolving component to perform out its typical physiological functions.

CHAPTER 3. WHAT IS CANCER

Cancer occurs when cells in the human body create irregularities and start to duplicate at anomalous quick rates. The outcome is the development of tumors in or on the surface of the body and organs. Tumors might be generous (not destructive) or threatening (harmful). Since ordinary cell improvement and duplication is a moderate procedure which is well controlled, it is evident when cells duplicate so rapidly.

Harmful tumors require quick regulation and treatment, as threatening developments may grow quickly and metastasize (spread all through the body) at a disturbing rate. Metastases are auxiliary tumors which can show up at any area all through the body, which is an immediate impact of disease spreading by means of blood and lymph hubs.

Cancer is only a term used to portray a vast assortment of sicknesses, affecting altogether different parts of the body in altogether different ways. There are two extensive classes into which all malignancy types can be isolated: hematological, which are blood-borne diseases and strong tumors, which are the developments depicted previously. Every kind of disease has an extraordinary name, more often than not originating from the range of the body which is fundamentally influenced. For instance, delicate tissue tumors are dangerous developments which happen inside the profound muscle or interfacing tissues all through the body. Melanoma is a sort of skin growth, which influences cells containing skin pigments.

As the main source of death in the United States, malignancy gets a gigantic measure of consideration from analysts and research healing centers devoted to deciding the cause and hunting down cures. Around one portion of men and 33% of ladies will build up some kind of malignancy amid their lifetime. Confidence is vital, be that as it may, as a great many individuals are presently living disease free on account of the endeavors of scientists and the donations of individuals over the world.

Everybody is at hazard for developing cancer; way of life changes, for example, stopping smoking and diminishing liquor admission could build a man's possibility of not building up a few tumors. Likewise, sound living and dietary decisions can also ensure that should a person get cancer they are more ready to battle it. It is additionally essential to see your doctor for examinations all the time keeping in mind the end goal to guarantee that legitimate testing should be possible if an issue is suspected.

Types of Cancer

Each year, over half a million people in the United States alone, die from cancer. But when we talk about this dreaded disease, it's important to keep in mind that several types of cancer exist. While the list virtually spans from A-to-Z, here are some of the most common ones:

Breast Cancer

Breast Cancer has become an epidemic among today's women. In fact, worldwide it's the most common type of cancer among women, and in the United States causes the second most cancer deaths among women. But not all the news is bad! Undergoing an annual mammogram can help to detect warning signs of the disease, such as changes in the structure of the breast tissue, and lumps that appear on the breast. The result is that women are generally able to detect the disease much earlier than they did in the past.

Researchers continue to learn more about the causes and effective treatments of breast cancer. They've learned that hormones and genes are the primary factors that determine a woman's likelihood of acquiring the disease. Physicians treat breast cancer based on the variety that the patient has acquired, and how broadly it has spread. Common treatments include hormonal therapy, chemotherapy, and radiation therapy.

Colon and Rectal Cancer

These two types of cancers are grouped together since they're involved in the digestion and excretion of food respectively. The two body parts form the large intestine. Cancer occurs in this system when tumors form on the large intestine's interior wall. It's important to note that the malignant tumors, rather than the benign ones, are the cancerous ones. But keep in mind that malignant tumors can become cancerous if you fail to remove them soon enough.

In some cases the cancer cells in the large intestine damage nearby or distant tissues and organs. For example, sometimes the cancer cells spread to distant organs, such as the lungs or liver. And the bad news is that once colon or rectal cancer spreads to other organs, it's improbable that the cancer victim will ever experience a complete recovery.

Worldwide, cancers of the colon and rectum are the third most common type of cancer. They're particularly common in Western countries, and in those nations where Western diets have become popular. This is mainly due to the high amount of processed and prepackaged food that people consume in those regions of the world.

Lung Cancer

As with all other types of cancer, the essence of lung cancer involves a problem with the normal process of cell growth. Basically, cells duplicate and divide abnormally, which ultimately results in a tumor. These tumors can be either benign (harmless), or malignant (harmful). Malignant tumors can grow out-of-control and can start affecting other tissues outside the lungs.

In fact, lung cancer is one of the most uncontrollable and deadly types of cancers. Why is that? It quickly begins spreading and infecting other parts of the body, such as the liver and brain. Also, the lung easily acquires tumors from cancer cells originating from other parts of the body. These are the reasons why treating lung cancer early is particularly important.

Different Types of Cancer Specialists and Their Qualifications

Cancer is one of those diseases that scare a patient to death even if he or she is far from it. In this regard, I need to remind you that cancer does not always mean death. There are different stages of cancer, and mostly the last-stage patients are beyond the recovery process. So, you should not shun away all hopes if one of your friends or family members gets diagnosed with cancer.

But you should never negate the seriousness of cancer. It is perhaps the trickiest and most complex disease in the world of medicine. This is the reason a cancer patient should rely on the combined care of different types of cancer specialists. What are these types? Let us have a look:

Different Types of Cancer Specialists

There are 3 ways of treating cancer: with surgery, with radiation, and with medicine. The type and stage of cancer decide whether a patient will need all these 3 types of treatments or not. Here is the list of the different cancer specialists you might need.

Surgical Oncologist: A surgical oncologist is a surgeon who specializes in diagnosing cancer with a biopsy. This oncologist can also treat this disease by removing cancer-infected tissues like tumors.

Radiation Oncologist: A radiation oncologist specializes in treating a cancer patient with radiation therapy. This process kills the cancer cells by sending high doses of radiation. Although this process affects the healthy cells around the cancer-infected ones, the cancer-infected cells die instantly and the healthy cells repair themselves back to normal.

Medical Oncologist: A medical oncologist is the most common cancer specialist. This specialist is the one who is in charge of a patient's frequent long-term checkups. A medical oncologist acts like an internist where he or she uses modern tools like internal medicine EHR software to treat a patient in a more organized, fast and efficient way. A medical oncologist is also in charge of immunotherapy, hormone therapy, and chemotherapy.

Important Qualifications of a Cancer Specialist

Now that you know about the different types, you should also have full knowledge about the important qualifications needed in a cancer specialist. Let us have a look:

Experience: As cancer is one of the most serious (and risky) diseases, the oncologist you are consulting must have a huge amount of experience in treating the specific type of cancer you have. You can ask him the number of patients he handles. As the minimal amount is tough to estimate, it is best to rely on his behavior and your gut feelings.

Board Certification: No matter which specialist you choose, he or she should have a board certificate. Board certification exams thoroughly test oncologists about their knowledge on cancer. Therefore, this certificate will act as a proof that the specialist you choose has a high skill-set.

Communication: This is perhaps the most important qualification your cancer specialist needs. A good oncologist tries to understand the pain of his patient. He can do this only by having good communication skills. He needs to talk less, and listen more. And he has to show that he cares for his patients.

Common Types of Cancer Treatments

In today's world, there are many different types of cancer - hundreds, actually. Medical professionals and researchers that focus on treating these diseases have conducted numerous studies and concluded that, for each individual type of cancer, there are at least one to two treatment methods that are most appropriate for alleviating the symptoms that are troublesome to the patient and slowing the progression of the illness. In this health guide, you will be introduced to several of the most common forms of treatments that are available for cancer patients.

Chemotherapy

One of the most common and most popular forms of treatment for cancer is chemotherapy. This is nothing more than a name given to medications that assist an individual in combating the effects of cancer. These medications are chemical based and work to completely kill off cancer cells within the body.

In addition to this, this type of cancer treatment has the capability of reducing the size of tumors in the body so that they may be eliminated by surgery, to enhance the overall effectiveness of other types of cancer treatment such as the popular radiation, and to overcome the body's overall resistance to cancerous cells. In addition to this, chemotherapy is said to enhance a patient's quality of living and comfort level while suffering from cancer.

Radiation Therapy

Radiation therapy is a popular type of cancer treatment. It has been established by medical professionals and other individuals that work directly with cancer patients that this type of therapy has the ability to reduce cancer cells, slow the progression of the duplication that occurs within cells in the body that have mutated, and even drastically reduce or completely eliminate tumors that may occur in the body due to the type of cancer that the patient is suffering from.

There are two basic types of radiation treatment for cancer. The first is external and is usually administered through the means of a beam. The second is internal and is normally administered through the means of injection in the area where the cancer cells are located.

Bone Marrow Transplant

Individuals that have certain types of cancer may benefit from the cancer treatment of a bone marrow transplant. Within the bone marrow, there are special cells that are identified by medical professionals as "Stem Cells". During a special surgical procedure, these cells are taken out of the bone marrow. The performing team of surgeons works to filter out the cells that they remove from the bone marrow.

Once the cells have been properly filtered, they may be issued back to the individual undergoing the treatment. In certain instances, individuals that undergo a bone marrow transplant will receive stem cells that have been filtered from other individuals prior to the surgical proceeding.

The Different Types of Cancer Clinical Trials

There are many different types of cancer clinical trials. Typically, it takes a long time to research various aspects of cancer. A clinical trial is the last part of the extensive research that has been performed when it comes to different types of cancers, cancer treatments, and other areas of importance when it comes to cancer.

These studies include a large variety of patients. The patients are subjected to prevention treatments, diagnostic tests, and even treatments that may assist in either the prevention of cancer as a whole, the resolution of symptoms associated with cancer, and slowing the overall progression of the disease in which they suffer. Here, you will be introduced to the different types of cancer clinical trials.

Screening Trials

Screening cancer clinical trials work to test new approaches and tests of identifying cancer in patients. The goal is to ensure that the cancer is identified prior to the symptoms of the disease setting in. Medical professionals, researchers, and specialists in certain branches of medicine will use a large assortment of diagnostic measures in order to identify cancer that is developing in the body.

The diagnostic tools may include imaging tests that use special technology in order to see inside and throughout the body. Basic laboratory tests are also utilized in screening trials. These include blood tests, tests that evaluate the urine and even biopsies that examine certain types of tissue and other components of the body. Genetic tests may also be used to identify biomarkers and any unusual DNA traits.

Prevention Trials

The prevention trials which are often identified as studies that are "chemoprevention", work to determine if taken certain actions will effectively reduce the possibility of developing cancer. There are two unique types of prevention trials. The first makes a determination as to if a person performing a certain type of action will prevent cancer development.

This is referred to as the "Action" trial. The "Agent" trial, on the other hand, is where the patient must engage in some type of ingestion such as taking medication and supplements in order to prevent the onset of cancer development in the body. These cancer clinical trials are usually quite extensive, and therefore take quite a bit of time in order to determine if they work or not.

Treatment Trials

Treatment trials are usually designated for cancer patients. These trials offer patients the ability to take a new medication, indulge in a new treatment, take part in alternative therapy, and many other treatments to see if it slows the progression of the disease in which they are suffering. Many of the treatments are not approved by the FDA but must undergo an evaluation period in order to reach that point. On the most part, participation is free and event-free, but there are some cases in which the patient may experience discomfort, or uncomfortable side effects and even allergic reactions. As you can see, there are many different cancer clinical trials available for patients that have cancer, their loved ones, and even those that want to prevent developing cancer.

Symptoms of Cancer

Cancer is a very general term, and so are the symptoms of cancer than I am going to recount. Many of the more than one hundred types of cancer demonstrate these symptoms; however, these are not confined to cancer alone. Other illnesses may also be signaled by these conditions this is why, once you experience them, you should pay your doctor a visit immediately.

Fatigue or a feeling of tiredness that is persistent is the most common symptoms for cancer especially to those already at the advanced stage. It is commonly caused by anemia, a state that is linked to certain types of cancers particularly to those types concerning the bowel.

Fever may also be a sign, although it is a very vague indicator because most diseases are related to it. If a fever is persistent or one that keeps coming back, it may indicate a weak immune system.

Weight loss is not always good news. If it happens unintentionally and significantly (about 10 pounds) with or without loss of appetite, then it might be something else. So does bowel changes. If you begin experiencing constipation, blood in stools, diarrhea, gas or anything unusual in you moving habit, it is just right to consult an expert.

A chronic cough may also be a symptom especially to those with lung cancer. Observe if it does not go away or if it keeps coming back and gets worse; especially if there are blood and mucus that comes with it.

Pain is another indicator but not for all types. Lung cancer patients may experience shoulder pain, those with colon cancer and ovarian cancer may feel lower back pain, and migraines are felt by those with brain cancer. Pain is felt particularly when cancer has spread.

Whichever of these symptoms you feel, it is best that you consult your doctor right away for early detection of any illnesses that may have caused them.

Techniques for checking a patient to confirm symptoms of cancer

Doctors may utilize different testing strategies to confirm if the patient is, in reality, experiencing cancer. In the case of visible tumors, a biopsy would demonstrate if the tumor is, in fact, dangerous or benign. Blood tests, Pap spread tests; stool and pee tests are a portion of alternate tests to check for particular proteins or different specialists that may demonstrate growth. A doctor may lead an endoscopy or colonoscopy to check for tumors inside a patient's stomach, colon or digestive system. An MRI output could likewise demonstrate tumors or variations from the norm in a patient and help the doctor find the correct position of disease.

There are many symptoms of cancer that manifest themselves but might end up getting confused with other diseases. Any change in routine should immediately be reported to a competent doctor and the necessary tests should be conducted to either get peace of mind or to catch cancer in the nascent stage itself.

CHAPTER 4. HOW CANCER DIAGNOSED

Cancer can send chills up anybody's spine. At whatever point a man hears the word coming from his/her specialist, a sentiment fear (and once in a while, impending doom) can wash over them. All things considered, who in their correct personality would feel cheerful about being determined to have a tumor?

Before giving any analysis of cancer to their patient, specialists would require him/her to experience a few tests. There are many research center testing administrations that specialists - and patients - depend on with respect to diagnosing and notwithstanding preventing cancer from happening. These research center testing administrations incorporate blood tests, tumor markers, and urinalysis.

The first of these clinical research center testing administrations are blood tests. These can recognize various red platelets, white platelets, and platelets in a patient's blood. Red platelets are for the transportation of oxygen to the diverse parts of the body, while platelets are the body's security from draining and wounding effectively. At the point when a blood test demonstrates that there is a bigger measure of white platelets in the body than common, it might imply that there is a disease. White platelets are in charge of battling any contamination that happens in the body.

In the event that specialists would depend on the results of blood tests alone, then there would be several specialists diagnosing patients with disease regardless of the possibility that the patient is just experiencing an episode of colds. This is the reason other research facility testing administrations are led with a specific end goal to ensure that the patient truly has the disease and not some different sickness.

The second test is a urinalysis. The body discharges distinctive substances, and by sifting or inspecting these substances display in the pee, specialists can check for any further indications of malignancy. Contrasted with the past two tests, tumor markers are as of now being utilized by specialists to screen the status of a patient's malignancy. Malignancy cells typically discharge certain substances that help specialists check if the disease has advanced or not. The therapeutic group is currently searching for methods for utilizing tumor markers to analyze, distinguish, and conceivably even treat cancer.

A cancer diagnosis can likewise be based on a patient's history and consequences of a physical examination. Be that as it may, these lab testing administrations give enough support at whatever point a specialist needs to educate his/her patient on the nearness, absence, and phase of cancer in the patient's body.

Breast Cancer

Three-quarters of patients with breast cancer not on factors that put them at increased risks for breast cancer, indicating that all risk factors appear well understood. Therefore, doctors have recommended that every woman must have a breast examination every year for a health care professional and should perform monthly self-examination have. A woman discovered a lump in your breast; you should inform your doctor immediately.

However, a lump in the women breasts is not a sign of cancer. Each breast is lumpy to some degree there is inflammation just before menstruation, breast enlargement, of course. In addition, some breast disease produces tumors, which can be confused with cancer. This non-cancerous growth includes cysts that are a thickening of breast tissue, milk is produced.

X-ray examination of breasts, this technique can increase the chances of success recognized in the treatment of tumors at an early stage before they are old enough to be felt. Although studies produced conflicting results on the effectiveness of this x-ray examination to reduce breast cancer risk and deaths, the ACS has recommended that women over 40 should have a mammogram check every year. However, a mammogram is unable to distinguish a benign from malignant tumors. The only way to make a correct diagnosis in the lymph suspect in the chest is a biopsy, a small operation that is part of the body or the tumor is removed and examined under the microscope to detect cancer cells in the humans' bodies.

If cancer is identified in the breasts, doctors try to determine if the malignant cells of the breast and the surrounding tissue, the serious and often fatal complications caused by metastases. The most common sites of metastases in patients with breast cancer are the lymph nodes under the arm. The absence or presence of cancer cells in lymph nodes help physicians to determine the extent to which cancer has progressed. Doctors remove several lymph nodes under the arm, to determine if cancer cells. This surgical procedure can result found lymphedema, it is a painful inflammation of the arm to fluid accumulation and a woman with an increased risk of infection. There is a new procedure called the sentinel lymph node biopsy, doctors use a less risky method to identify and remove a sentinel lymph node, a single ganglion cell cancer in the first trip. If the sentinel nodes contain the cancer cells, cancer has not spread across the chest and the women are saved more extensive surgery.

CHAPTER 5. NATURAL REMEDY FOR CANCER

In the recent years, there has been an increasing trend towards developing alternative natural cures for cancer. It is been increasingly advised by oncologists and physicians practicing general medicine that the cancer patients must incorporate the intake of a few supplements into their regular diet as they are crucial to maintaining their good health and overall well-being.

There are three supplements that act as nature's cures in healing the effects of cancer. It has been seen that a high potency mineral and multivitamins offer adequate levels of the essential minerals and all other vitamins. It is necessary to go for a high potency multiple that needs to be consumed at least twice daily. The dosage should be around two to three tablets. Green drinks are said to be high on dehydrated wheat grass and barley grass. These contain algae which serve as a rich source of spirulina or chlorella. These are also referred to as green superfoods as they are high on chlorophyll and carotenes, both of which are known as cancer-fighting phytochemicals.

Doctors also advise their patients' fish oil that has been manufactured by a pharmaceutical company. Fish oil is a rich source of omega-3 fatty acids. The long chain omega fatty acids are also alternatively referred to as DHA or docosahexaenoic acid and EPA or eicosapentaenoic acid. These acids form at least 60% of the total weight of the fish oil. These supplements are practically devoid of heavy metals, lipid peroxides, and environmental contaminants.

Apart from these foundational supplements, a number of other specific natural medicines can also be used. A couple of natural cancer fighters include maitake mushroom extract and proteolytic enzymes. The extract of the maitake mushroom, also known as the grifola from dosa, serves as one of the best natural cures for cancer. This extract is naturally rich in immunity-enhancing compounds which are also known as beta-glucans. These are known for their cancer-fighting properties.

Proteolytic enzymes are known for their numerous benefits, especially as one of the natural remedies to cure cancer. It assists in the absorption of protein. These comprise papain or papaya enzyme, pancreatic proteases chymotrypsin, Serratia peptidase, bromelain, and trypsin. It has been proven by consistent clinical studies that these enzymes help in improving the condition of cancer patients and have a positive effect on their quality of life. They also have a fine safety profile.

However, these should not be used a couple of days prior to a surgery or after it as they might increase the chances of bleeding.

My "Past Budwig" Recipe

As a result of the adjustments in agribusiness, I propose this updated 21st-century version of the Budwig Protocol:

6 ounces refined dairy

4 tablespoons grew and ground chia or flax

1 tablespoon flaxseed oil

1 teaspoon turmeric powder

1/4 teaspoon dark pepper

Combine every one of the fixings in bowl or blender and expand once day by day.

The Foods You Should Be Eating to Cure Your Cancer Naturally

In the event that you are battling tumor, it is imperative to be exceptionally strict about each nourishment thing that you put in your mouth. The purpose behind this is with regards to tumor, there are two sorts of foods, those that reinforce the body with a specific end goal to murder carcinogenic cells and those that nourish tumor cells.

In this sub-chapter, we will talk about the foods boost your immune system so that the dangerous cells will cease to exist. These are the malignancy slaughtering nourishments.

Dark leafy greens are a standout amongst the most capable foods that anybody battling tumor can devour. Nourishments, for example, collards, spinach, romaine lettuce, broccoli, kale, and parsley are stuffed with supplements that have a stunning recuperating impact on the body. The reason is on account of these foods contain a lot of carotenoids. Carotenoids scour the body looking for harmed and infected cells.

When they come into contact with these cells, they obliterate them. It is imperative to note, in any case, that expending these things crude, in their regular frame, will give your body substantially more quick mending. Cooking these carotenoid-rich foods down to a soft consistency obliterates the recuperating influence in the nourishments.

Antioxidant rich foods are likewise critical. Cell reinforcements are found in other plant-based nourishments, basically those which contain a lot of vitamin C and vitamin E. Nourishments, for example, blueberries, strawberries, lemons and limes fall into this classification. Obviously, there are numerous others. Green tea is additionally high in cell reinforcements and is an awesome drink to expend various circumstances for the duration of the day.

You likewise need to devour nourishments which are high in fiber. High fiber foods waste to travel through the body inside a sensible measure of time. When you don't have high measures of fiber in your eating regimen, the waste stays in your body and your body will get to be distinctly dangerous as the sustenance spoils within you. You cannot recuperate your body on the off chance that it is toxic.

Flax seeds are an incredible wellspring of fiber, as well as these little seeds contain capable tumor slaughtering supplements too. Mixing up flax seeds and placing it in your smoothies, on your oat or over your plates of mixed greens at every dinner will do ponders for both your wellbeing and your assimilation. Malignancy can just form and flourish in a harmful and acidic environment. Understand that waste out of your body with the goal that you are not making your body more poisonous. Increment your fiber intake right away!

It is additionally imperative to expend bunches of crisp clean water. In the event that you increment your fiber admission without expanding your water utilization, you will get stopped up. On the off chance that you are obstructed, the waste is not leaving your body. Endeavor to drink half of your body weight in ounces of water every day.

While battling cancer, it is critical to be aware of each and every thing that you put into your mouth. As expressed over, the times of eating unwittingly should end on the off chance that you are not kidding about overcoming this disease.

A Natural and Nutritious Diet to Support Cancer Medicines and Treatments

There is no denying the fact that a highly nutritious diet is essential during a battle against cancer. It has been observed that cancer patients who maintain a highly nutritional diet succeed in overcoming the threat of infections and also recover from any illness much faster. They are also able to better withstand the side effects of any kind of therapy. A nutritional diet is thus one of the much-advised treatments to cancer.

Be it cancer or any other disease, physicians and health experts agree that a healthy diet serves as the cure of all diseases. It is necessary to work on the eating habits of the patients who are currently undergoing treatment such as radiation or chemotherapy. Hence, it's significant to ensure that they:

Drink at least six to eight glasses of water on a regular basis which will keep them hydrated

Have 450 to 600 ml of homemade and fresh vegetable juice along with their food. This can also be alternatively be made a kind of mid-morning breakfast or a sort of a juice break

Consume a high protein drink such as a smoothie containing about 25g to 30g of whey protein at least once or even twice a day. This can serve as an alternative to breakfast and also as a mid-afternoon snack.

Opt for small meals but at regular intervals during the course of the day in place of heavy meals.

Make use of additional seasonings, flavors and spices so that the food tastes good and thus tempts them to finish off the serving

Stay away from flavorings that make the food exceptionally sweet or bitter as prolonged cancer treatment can alter the taste of the food completely and make it different.

Consume small bites at a time and chew the food well rather than gulping it down.

Eat moist and soft food items such as yams, bananas, brown rice instead of opting for dry and hard food items such as hard candies, cereals, and crackers.

Though radiation and chemotherapy are the most widely used treatments for cancer, many doctors' advice natural remedies to cure cancer these days. The high dose of medicines and therapies need to be supplemented with a rich and nutritious diet into order to ensure that the treatments work effectively. Therefore it is absolutely necessary that a proper diet is formed and implemented as it is one of the best natural cures for cancer.

How to Prevent Cancer Naturally With Specific Foods

Cancer has become a frightening specter of murder, cruel and indiscriminate towards his victims. Nowadays, cancer has become the top killer not only in developed countries but also in developing countries. Cancer development as it is now inseparable from the changing pattern of human life including diet which consumes a lot of junk food like fast food carbonated drinks like soft drinks, smoking and so forth.

Food or what we eat plays a very important role in the occurrence of disease, disease progression, and severity of a disease. Cancer is one disease or the changes that can be caused by the wrong diet and not pay attention to nutritional balance eaten daily. We should pay attention to nutritional balance and the balance of nature in consuming foods daily. Human must consume food in accordance with the menu or nutritional balance between carbohydrate, protein, fat, vitamins and minerals.

There are several things that must be considered so that we can avoid or be cured of cancer that may arise in our body because of our wrong diet. First, only consume fresh foods like vegetables, fruits, and meat. Try to only eat the flesh of fish just because the meat of cows, goats, pigs and chickens contain fat that are not good for human body. Second, you should avoid consuming cow's milk because it is not suitable for humans. Cow's milk in the human body will quickly clot and cannot be digested properly, so ended up going to cause allergies and even osteoporosis. Replace your milk immediately with soy milk. Also avoid other dairy products like cheese, yogurt or other milk products. Third, avoid bad eating habits such as consuming alcohol, soft drinks, coffee, tea, and smoking. Only drink water that contains minerals as much as possible because water also has the function to remove toxins and cleanse the body and digestive system.

Do not forget to always enjoy life with a cheerful and happy, because if you feel happy then your body's endurance will be increased in order to combat a variety of disturbances in your body including the fight against disease and cancer.

Natural Prevention of Collagen Degradation and Enzyme-Blocking Therapy

Lysine as a Natural Enzyme Block

The activation of this collagen-dissolving component prompts to the improvement of forceful sicknesses, for example, tumor and microbial diseases. Aside from that, this instrument assumes a critical part in all ailments that advance to cutting edge stages. Each remedial probability that will end instrument or even back off will hence be a standout amongst the most vital achievements the field of medicine.

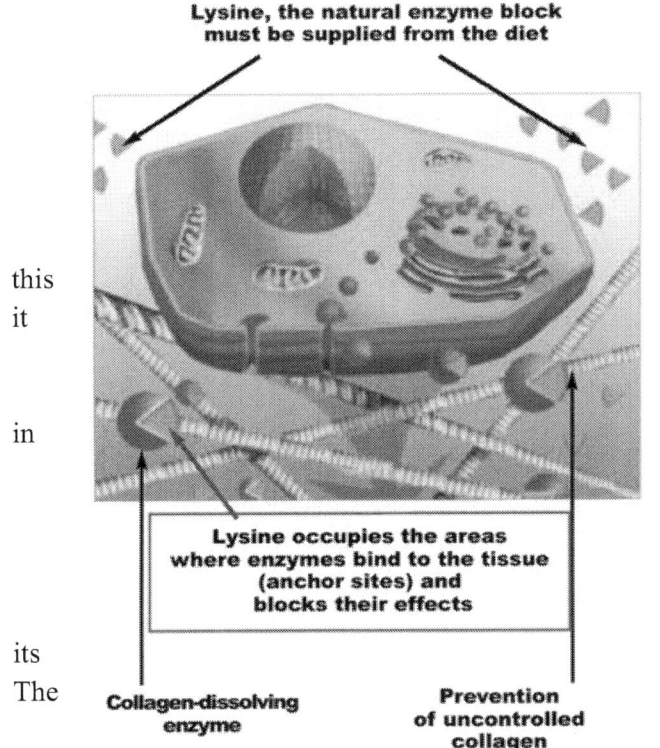

Nature itself provides us with two huge groups of atoms that can square collagen absorption and dissolving activities. primary gathering is the body's characteristic enzymatic piece that can stop the activity of collagen-processing proteins in no time flat. The second gathering is the catalyst blocking substances that originate from our eating routine or as the dietary supplement. An essential one in this gathering is the normal amino corrosive L-lysine. At the point when lysine is provided in an adequate sum as a dietary supplement, it can obstruct the stay locales in the connective tissue that collagen-processing chemicals use to append themselves to the tissue. In this way, lysine prevents these catalysts from wildly crumbling connective tissue.

This is represented on the following page: while the cells still create elevated amounts of collagen-processing chemicals, within the sight of lysine these proteins are no longer successful in separating collagen. Along these lines, the uncontrolled annihilation of collagen and connective tissue structure can be anticipated. Along these lines, the spread of infections can be backed off or ceased**Lysine Is the Most Effective Natural Way to Block Collagen-DigestinEnzymes**

The Lysine

Remarkable Value of Every body is dialect.

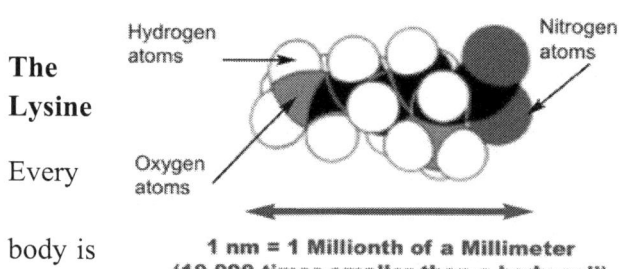

To date, approximately twenty known amino acids make every one of the proteins in our bodies. These building pieces of life capacity like the letters of the letters in order. Our body utilizes different mixes of amino acids to make multitudinous organic words (peptides) and sentences (proteins). Isolate amino acids (letters) likewise have vital "individual" metabolic capacities, and lysine is a prime case.

The cells of the body can create most amino acids themselves. These amino acids are called insignificant. Be that as it may, there are nine known amino acids that our body can't create, and they must be provided through the eating regimen. These amino acids are called basic (required forever).

Inside the gathering of fundamental amino acids, lysine assumes an also essential part as vitamin C does inside the vitamin assemble. The day by day prerequisite of lysine outperforms that of all other amino acids. Among its many capacities, lysine is likewise the essential building piece of the amino corrosive carnitine, which is vital for vitality digestion system in each cell.

The way that the human body can store a lot of this amino corrosive is evidence enough of its significance for our wellbeing. Around 25% of collagen, the richest and imperative basic particle of bones, skin, vein dividers, and every other organ comprises of two amino acids, lysine, and proline. As the rundown on the following page appears, a man measuring 70 kg (155 lb.) has around 500 g (1.1 lb.) of lysine put away in the body in all circumstances.

Taking vast amounts of lysine won't bring about unfavorable impacts. Our digestion system knows about taking care of a lot of lysines, and it will basically discharge the atoms that are not utilized. Or maybe, the inverse is, for the most part, the case: Almost all individuals experience the ill effects of an incessant lack of lysine.

The Balance between Collagen Dissolving Enzymes and Lysine

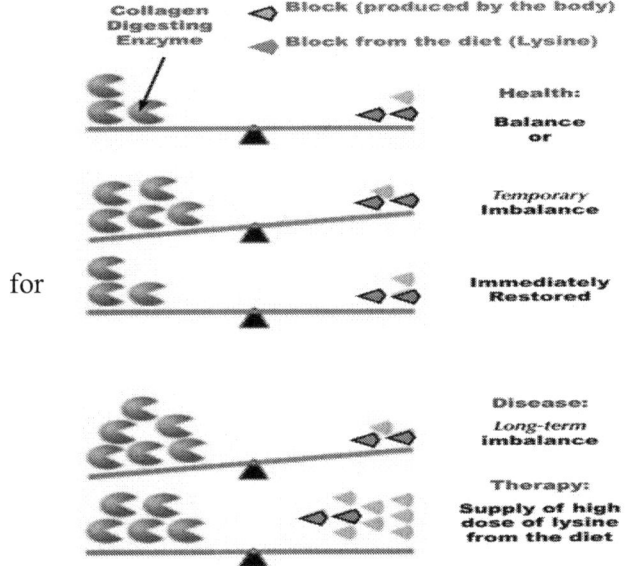

We have effectively discovered that compound movement can be obstructed with the body's own particular particles and with those provided through the eating routine, for example, lysine. The bodies own Particular Square (enzymatic inhibitor) is the primary line of barrier that guarantees assures the balance among the body's systems and holds them under wraps. In the representation, the catalyst square delivered by the body is spoken to by green bolts. Lysine particles have a similar capacity however are the second lines of barrier, prepared to venture in when the body's own particular frameworks are deficient. The lysine piece can't overshoot its objective, notwithstanding when taken in high sums, for example, 4 oz. then again 8 oz. a day.

A second important fact shown in the outline is the harmony between the collagen-dissolving instrument (red) and its blocking system (green) amid affliction and wellbeing. In ordinary conditions these frameworks are in impeccable adjust. At the point when "police cells" are meandering through the body, the balance is exasperates. Yet, the sound body then reestablishes the balance within moments.

In growth and other already portrayed maladies, this balance gets to be distinctly upset for the collagen-dissolving instrument. Since the characteristic cell instruments can't adequately obstruct the collagen-breaking down process, a high-measurements dietary supplement of lysine is the main conceivable treatment to stop or to back off this procedure. The objective of this treatment is to revise the disturbed adjust with a long haul high convergence of lysine to square deterioration.

Collagen Digesting Enzymes and Their Blocks in Disease and Health

Successful Use of Enzyme Blocks in Cancer Therapy

Efficient control of the spread of an ailment by collagen dissolving protein pieces has been effective with a few infections. This is particularly imperative in maladies for which customary pharmaceutical has no preventive or recuperating treatments yet. This incorporates the types of cancer illustrated on the following page.

To date many reviews have set up that a high-dose supply of vitamin C, vitamin E, beta-carotene, and other dietary supplements can keep a few forms of cancer. There is more data regarding this matter in the writing recorded in the book index. A supply of vitamins in high measurements shapes the reason for each present cancer therapy.

Vitamin treatment has made restorative progress in hormone-autonomous types of cancer; though in hormone subordinate types of cancer the characteristic treatments have been either barely compelling or not fruitful.

Presently, surprisingly we have available to us a viable type of a characteristic treatment, in view of obstructing the enzymatic demolition of collagen. As found in the case of ovulation, these collagen-dissolving chemicals are specifically initiated by hormones; in this manner the utilization of lysine in high doses can be successful in treating all types of cancer.

Enzyme-blocking Therapy for Cancer

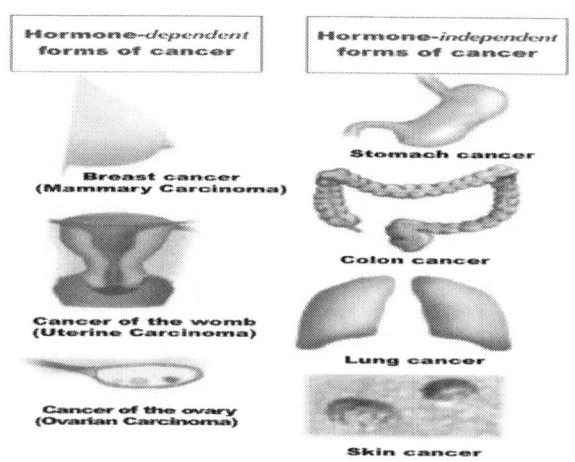

The Use of Lysine in Other Serious Diseases

The therapeutic applications for lysine in the battle against ailment are not confined to cancer. It can be utilized as a part of the common treatment of numerous different infections for which conventional medication has not yet found an answer. Diseases that can be treated with high measurements of lysine are recorded in the table on the following page.

In atherosclerosis, lysine can stop the spread and development of stores (atherosclerotic plaques) in the veins of the heart and mind. In the meantime, with the assistance of vitamins and other dietary supplements, a characteristic mending procedure of the blood vessel dividers can begin.

In irresistible diseases brought on by infections, for example, influenza, herpes, and AIDS; or created by microbes, for example, lung, inward ear, and bladder diseases; lysine can stop or back off a forceful spread of contamination. A mix of high measurements of vitamin C and other dietary supplements can bring extra advantages.

Indeed, even on account of perpetual irritation of the stomach, digestion tracts, joints, and bones the utilization of lysine can hold the aggravation under control. Successful treatment of constant aggravation includes the utilization of high measurements of lysine joined with other vital dietary supplements.

Indeed, even exceptionally regular hypersensitive issues, for example, feed fever, neurodermatitis, or vex rash, can benefit by the utilization of lysine, which can alleviate the sickness or counteract it. In these cases I likewise suggest consolidating lysine with vitamin C and other dietary supplements.

Conventional Cancer Therapy - a Dead-End Street

When you have achieved this point in the book, you will without a doubt ask yourself, "Is the therapeutic world on the wrong track with its cancer therapy?" My answer would be, "Yes!"

The routine treatment of cancer includes surgery, radiation treatment, and particularly chemotherapy. None of these treatments has been demonstrated to augment the life of a patient. This implies these treatments have been utilized for a considerable length of time despite the fact that doctors realize that it won't mend the malady and will frequently even quicken it.

Always compelled by the pharmaceutical business, patients are offered no alternatives until they consent to chemotherapy. Chemotherapy implies harming the cells. The pharmaceutical business offers this cell harm with the contention that it will harm the cancer cells. What they don't tell patients is that the various cells of the body are harmed too. In this way, chemo-harming of the bone marrow - where fresh recruit's cells are created will prompt to iron deficiency and expanded defenselessness to diseases. Chemo - harming of the mucous film cells of the gastrointestinal tract will prompt to the looseness of the bowels and intestinal bleeding.

The damage to hair follicles prompts to an extraordinary loss of hair. Rather than fortifying the body's safe framework to battle cancer, the chemotherapy will paralyze it.

Chemotherapy's symptoms require the extra utilization of other, new pharmaceuticals, for example, anti-infection agents, plasma substitution drugs, painkillers, cortisone, and some more. The most recent weeks or months of life for the patients undergoing cancer therapy are an Eldorado for the pharmaceutical business.

Cancer - No Longer a Death Warrant

Without precedent for the historical backdrop of pharmaceutical plainly:

Not just tumor and some chose infections, additionally basically all known illnesses utilize the collagen-dissolving component to spread through the body.

The collagen-dissolving component assumes an essential part in the development of plaques in cutting edge atherosclerosis.

The utilization of high-measurement lysine or lysine subordinates can back off or stop the spread of practically every malady. The way that lysine in blend with vitamin C can balance out the connective tissue in the body is a restorative leap forward in the control of numerous ailments so far considered hopeless.

The across the board utilization of this treatment will prompt to an achievement in the battle against malignancy, irresistible illnesses - including AIDS and all different ailments.

Principles of Natural Therapies

Vitamin C and Lysine: Key Molecules of Health

Cell Health considers vitamin C (ascorbic corrosive) and the amino corrosive L-lysine as the most imperative normal substances. Their lack in people can prompt to brokenness. There are two essential reasons why practically every individual experiences an insufficiency of these phone calculates: the human body can't deliver them, and our cutting edge dietary propensities can't give them in adequate sums. The outcome is that lone peripheral measures of these substances are found in the body.

All diseases flourish with an absence of vitamin C and lysine to spread through the body. This is identified with the unprecedented estimation of these substances for the body's connective tissue. We can compress this as takes after:

Lysine hinders the devastation of the connective tissue by forestalling enzymatic processing of collagen particles. In the meantime the amino corrosive lysine is a segment of collagen and it is utilized for making the collagen in the body.

Vitamin C empowers the creation of the connective tissue and is basic for its ideal structure, lack of vitamin C prompts to tissue shortcoming and in the long run to scurvy. Then again, an ideal supply of vitamin C guarantees ideal creation of collagen and flexible fiber particles and adds to having solid connective tissue in the body.

Vitamin C and Lysine - Effective Protection of the Connective Tissue

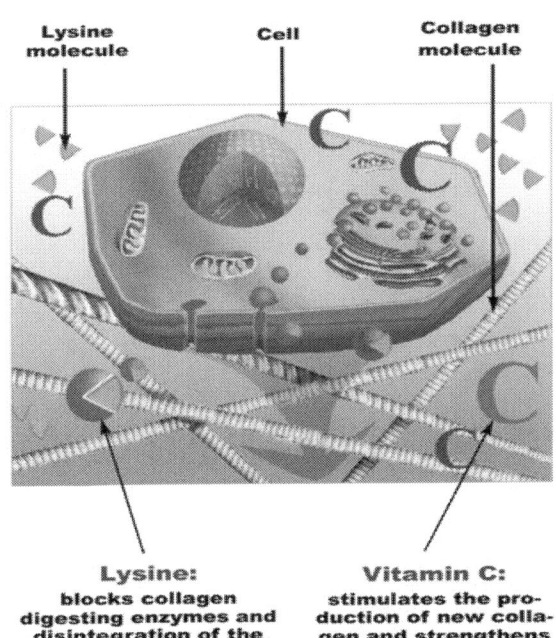

Collagen Production - A Key to Disease Prevention and Control

Ideal creation of collagen particles is the precondition for control of forceful illnesses. The photo on the following page demonstrates a muscle cell of the blood vessel divider. These blood vessel divider cells, among other physiological errands, need to deliver enough collagen particles to keep up the blood vessel divider solid and versatile. For ideal collagen generation they require three noteworthy supplements:

Vitamin C, which controls the collagen generation from the cell core's product. Collagen atoms, which twist around each other like a twilled rope, can't achieve theoptimal structure basic for organic movement and soundness of collagen without the nearness of vitamin C. This ideal organic compliance is accomplished when "concoction" connects appropriately interface collagen strands, balancing out the whole structure. These extensions are shaped with oxygen and hydrogen particles - the alleged "Goodness bunches" - , which stay particular lysine and proline atoms in collagen. This "hydroxylation" process is catalyzed by vitamin C.

Lysine, which is a building piece of the chain of amino acids that frame collagen strands. Since our body can't create its own particular lysine, each and every lysine particle must be provided through the eating routine or from dietary supplements.

Proline, which is another vital amino corrosive part of collagen. Our body can deliver it, however just in constrained sums. In individuals with long haul or forceful infections joined by the enzymatic demolition of tissue collagen, the body's ability to create proline can be depleted. This regularly prompts to an inadequacy of this vital amino corrosive.

Amino Acids Proline and Lysine Are Building Blocks of Collagen

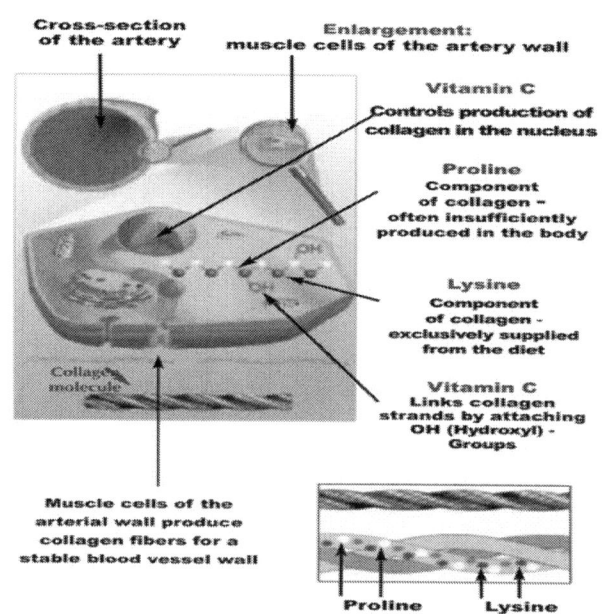

Healthful Supplementation with Proline, Lysine and Vitamin C

Adjusted amounts of L-proline, L-lysine, and vitamin C are fundamental for ideal generation of collagen atoms. Lysine is a fundamental amino corrosive that must be given in our eating routine. In spite of the fact that proline can be combined in our body, its amounts may not be adequate for particular body needs. An extra admission of proline can profit individuals with an expanded requirement for this amino acid.

Proline, Lysine and the "Principle of the Weakest Link"

Any framework is just in the same class as its weakest part. This not just applies to a container loaded with water, additionally to the way our body produces collagen. Give me a chance to give you a case of a circumstance when proline is the weakest connection in the collagen generation chain. This would imply that this amino corrosive is the most required. In such conditions collagen can't be delivered in ideal sums regardless of the possibility that the supply of lysine and vitamin C is adequate. For this situation, more proline must be given. This is imperative, on the grounds that traditional medication still mistakenly trusts that the body itself can deliver any measure of proline and that an outside supply is not required. Taking after this wrong observation regularly brings lethal outcomes.

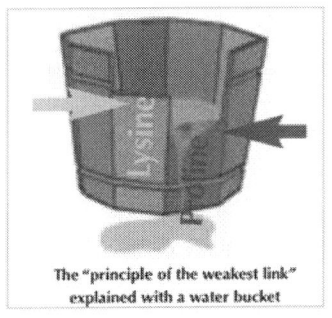

The "principle of the weakest link" explained with a water bucket

Cellular Health

Cell Health underlines the significance of supplement supplementation for ideal wellbeing. Vitamins, minerals, follow components and amino acids are fundamental in upgrading cell work in the body. These supplements mix together in cell digestion system like artists like artists in the symphony. The prerequisites for specific supplements differ from individual to individual and they generally rely on upon the hereditary make-up, ways of life or health conditions.

When all is said in done we have to ensure that supplements, for example, vitamin C and amino acids lysine and proline are given in ideal sums. These supplements are the building pieces of collagen, elastin and different segments of the connective tissue in our body. They likewise incorporate connective tissue establishing components, for example, chondroitin sulfate and different glycosaminoglycans. These supplements are basic for legitimate structure and ideal capacity of this tissue manufactures and pastes all cells together and shapes body organs. These supplements ought to be added to your eating routine steadily so your body has room schedule-wise to conform and react to them.

Today traditional prescription is in a phase of disappointment. Notwithstanding a huge number of dollars spent on pharmacological research, growth, coronary ailment, and other normal medical issues continue spreading like out of control fire. The main reason that these sicknesses are not controlled is that their actual causes have not been comprehended or have been disregarded; subsequently no compelling, ordinary treatment is accessible.

CHAPTER 6. CARE GIVING FOR YOUR LOVED ONE

In the event that you are watching over a friend or family member with cancer, you are a "caregiver." You may not consider yourself a guardian. You may perceive what you're doing as something common: dealing with somebody you adore. Still, for some individuals, mind giving isn't simple. However, there are numerous things you can do to make it less troublesome.

This part is intended to help you, the caregiver. It is loaded with tips from the expert oncology social specialists at Cancer Care, a national charitable association that has inhabited with tumor and their guardians for over 70 years. Our social workers individuals adapt to the passionate and pragmatic difficulties of cancer.

Perused this section straight through, or refer to various subsections as you need them. A few segments may not have any significant bearing to your circumstance. Utilize this section in the way works best for you. Make certain to converse with your cherished one regularly about what he or she feels would be generally useful.

In addition, investigate the rundown of extra assets we've given above of this booklet. Here, you'll discover great idea and tips of an assortment of associations, including Cancer Care that can reduce the trouble of being a guardian for somebody with malignancy.

The Role of the Caregiver

Caregivers give vital passionate and physical watch over a man with cancer. Regularly, caregivers are relatives or companions. They may live adjacent or far from the individual they look after.

There are a wide range of approaches to be a caregiver. Care giving can mean helping your cherished one with day by day exercises, for example, getting to the specialist or preparing meals. It can likewise mean helping the individual adapt to sentiments that surface amid this time.

The kind of bolster that a parental figure gives will be diverse to every individual. All in all, care giving assignments fall into three classifications:

Medical

Emotional and

Practical

This part gives numerous cases of things in each of these classes that caregivers can do to offer assistance.

Helping to Manage Your Loved One's Treatment

Sometimes, a man determined to have growth feels overpowered and may require somebody to help him or her deal with treatment choices. On the other hand, he or she may need somebody there to listen to the specialist's guidelines. A man getting treatment may require a caregiver's assistance in overseeing reactions or taking prescription or medication.

Here are some approaches to deal with your loved one's treatment:

Accumulate data

Find out about your loved one's diagnosis and conceivable treatment options. One great place to begin is by asking the specialist or medical caretaker what assets he or she suggests. There are additionally numerous dependable sites and malignancy associations that can give precise, a la mode restorative data.

Go to medicinal appointments together. Prior to a visit with the specialist, record any inquiries you two might want to inquire. Bring a note pad or compact voice recorder, so you can monitor the specialist's answers and allude to them later.

In the event that you have to talk with the human services group without your adored one present, get some answers concerning the guidelines of the Health Insurance Portability and Accountability Act (HIPAA). This law gives patients more noteworthy access to their own restorative records and more control over how their wellbeing data is utilized. Your cherished one should give composed authorization, by marking an assent shape, before specialists can impart data to you about his or her medicinal treatment.

Things to ask the Doctor

Here are a few inquiries you or your love one might need to ask the specialist:

What are the objectives of treatment?

How long will treatment last?

Do you have any composed data about this treatment?

What are the symptoms of this treatment?

Are there any approaches to oversee reactions?

How would we know whether a symptom is sufficiently serious to call you?

Are there whatever other treatment choices?

Are there any clinical trials we ought to know about?

What is the most ideal approach to tell you when we have inquiries regarding treatment?

Figure out how to help with physical care

Depending upon how they are feeling, individuals experiencing cancer and treatment may require help with an extensive variety of exercises they would ordinarily do themselves, for example, showering or dressing. Request that your adored one let you know how he or she needs you to help with these errands.

Get some information about unique guidelines

Check with the specialist or medical attendant to see whether there are particular guidelines you ought to know about. For instance, are there any tips for dealing with a specific reaction or does an uncommon eating regimen should be taken after treatment? Keep the specialist's telephone number in a place that is anything but difficult to discover on the off chance that you have questions.

Find out about associations that assistance with medical care

In the event that you require help dealing with some of your loved one's therapeutic needs, ask your specialist or clinic social laborer about neighborhood home wellbeing offices. These agencies may send attendants to the home to give medications, screen fundamental signs or change gauzes, for example. Home wellbeing offices can likewise send mind suppliers who go to other individual needs, for example, showering, and dressing, cooking or cleaning.

Giving Emotional Support

Experiencing growth is regularly depicted as a passionate exciting ride, with many high points and low points. As a parental figure, you may see your cherished one experience an extensive variety of feelings. While this can be troublesome for both of you, your eagerness to listen and offer support will have any kind of effect.

It is difficult to watch somebody you think about experience such a large number of troublesome feelings. There are things you can do; in any case, to help both of you cope with the situation:

Listen to your loved one.

It is imperative to listen without judging or "cheerleading." We are regularly enticed to state "you will be fine" when we hear unnerving or pitiful musings. Be that as it may, essentially listening to those sentiments can be a standout amongst the most imperative commitments you make.

Do what works

Consider how you've helped each other feel better during a troublesome time in the past. Was a fun excursion an accommodating diversion? Then again do you two incline toward calm circumstances and discussion? Do whatever works for you both, and don't be hesitant to have a go at something new.

Bolster your loved one's treatment choices

While you might be in a position to share basic decision, at last it is the other individual's body and soul that bear the effect of the cancer and its treatment.

Get data about support groups

Joining a support group allows your loved one to converse with others adapting with cancer and realize what they do to oversee troublesome feelings. Here and there, care groups are driven by social laborers or guides. Approach a healing center social specialist for a referral or contact Cancer Care.

In the event that it's required, proceed with your bolster when treatment is over. This can be a passionate time for some individuals. In spite of being calmed that the cancer is going away (stopped developing or vanished), a man may feel frightened that it will return. The finish of treatment likewise implies fewer gatherings with the social insurance group, on which the individual may have depended for support.

Adapting To Difficult Feelings

Individuals with cancer frequently feel emotions, for example,

Sadness

Sadness can go back and forth during treatment. For a few people, it can be more consistent or last more.

Outrage

For instance, individuals can be irate about the way treatment and symptoms make them feel or about the progressions their diagnosis has made in their lives.

Stress

Cancer can be a standout amongst the most unpleasant occasions a man encounters. Normal stresses incorporate dread of treatment not working, of cancer returning or spreading, and of conceivably losing control over one's life and future. Different stresses that existed before the cancer diagnosis, for example, work or monetary concerns, can add to the anxiety.

Suggest an oncology social specialist or instructor to give accommodating data and support. In the event that you think your loved one may require extra bolster adapting to his or her feelings amid this time, recommend talking with an expert who can help, for example, an oncology social worker.

Helping Your Loved One with Practical Matters

Notwithstanding assisting with restorative and passionate concerns, guardians regularly help by going up against numerous viable assignments. Sometime in the not so distant future to-day exercises parental figures can do incorporate running errands, contributing with family unit tasks, get ready suppers and assisting with tyke mind.

Since cancer can likewise put a gigantic strain on a family's accounts, caregivers are regularly left with the assignment of overseeing monetary issues, as well. Luckily, there are numerous assets accessible to offer assistance.

Here are a few tips for finding monetary help for costs identified with cancer:

Survey your cherished one's protection approaches to comprehend what's secured. Your insurance agency can relegate a caseworker who can clarify what administrations and medications the arrangement does and doesn't cover and answer any inquiries. Caseworkers work for protection and different sorts of offices. They help customer's access assets and administrations. He or she can likewise clarify any out-of-system advantages the strategy may offer, for example, restorative administrations from specialists not on your protection arrange.

Comprehend what your loved one is qualified for. A few sorts of help for individuals with cancer are required by law. These projects are called qualifications - government programs that give money related and other guide to individuals in specific gatherings, for example, those with tumor. A healing center or group social specialist can guide you to the legislative organizations that direct these projects.

Request offer assistance. On the off chance that you require help with healing facility charges, address a money related instructor in the doctor's facility's business office. He or she can work out a regularly scheduled installment arrange. On the off chance that your cherished one hopes to come up short on cash, or has as of now, converse with his or her leasers. Numerous landowners, utilities, and home loan organizations will work out an installment arrange before an emergency creates. Connecting for help at an opportune time is generally useful.

Monitoring Important Papers

Many individuals think that it's supportive to keep all records or printed material in one place. This will make things simpler in the event that you have addresses or are attempting to prepare.

Essential archives include:

Copies of therapeutic records

Prescription data

Health protection records

Disability protection

Long-term mind protection

Annuities

Social Security records

Veterans benefits

Bank articulations

Wills

Health mind intermediary

Power of lawyer

Apply for money related offer assistance. For some individuals, expensive cancer pharmaceuticals represent a financial challenge. Luckily, there are many projects to help qualified people get drugs for nothing or requiring little to no effort.

Dealing with a friend or family member can be a positive experience

For instance, a few people say that care giving reinforces their relationship. In any case, it can likewise be extremely upsetting. Numerous parental figures say it regularly feels like an all day work. Mind giving can be considerably additionally difficult in the event that you have numerous different obligations, such as working, bringing up youngsters or administering to your own wellbeing.

Sometimes, caregivers tend to put their own needs and emotions aside. It is vital, however, for you to take great care of yourself. This will make the experience of dealing with another person less upsetting for you.

Staying Healthy

Caregivers invest a great deal of energy caring for the soundness of their friends and family. This regularly implies the parental figure invests less energy concentrating on his or her needs, for example, eating admirably and working out. However dealing with your own physical wellbeing is an imperative piece of care giving.

Here are a few tips for watching over your health:

Stay active: Specialists prescribe practicing for no less than 30 minutes every day. Exercises can include strolling rapidly, running or riding a bicycle. Remember that you don't need to set aside a ton of time to work out - you can work it into your day. For instance, take the stairs rather than the lift, or stop your auto more distant away than you ordinarily do.

Focus on what you're eating: Keeping a balanced eating routine is an imperative piece of dealing with yourself. Include products of the soil in your dinners. Nuts, yogurt and nutty spread sandwiches are simple snacks with heaps of protein that will keep your vitality level up. Pack snacks in the event that you know you will be with your cherished one at the specialist's office or the hospital all day.

Get enough rest: Care giving can be sincerely and physically depleting. You may get yourself more drained than expected. Attempt to get enough rest, and take naps when you require them.

Rest regularly: As a caregiver, you may find that it is difficult to relax, regardless of the possibility that you have time for it. Profound breathing, thinking or delicate extending activities can help reduce stress.

Stay aware of your own checkups, screenings and medications: Your health is extremely profitable. Remain on top of your physical checkups, and have a framework for remembering to take any medicines you have to remain healthy.

Getting Emotional Support

Care giving is diligent work that can influence your passionate prosperity. Taking care of yourself incorporates coping to your very own large number sentiments that surface as you administer to your adored one. Many individuals feel more passionate than expected when they are adapting to a friend or family member's tumor. This is normal.

You can't make troublesome sentiments go away, however there are things you can improve.

Here are a few tips for adapting to the enthusiastic effect of your loved one's cancer:

Take a break. On the off chance that conceivable, take some time out for yourself consistently. Regardless of the possibility that it's only for a couple of minutes, accomplishing something you appreciate can help you energize. For instance, listening to unwinding music or going out for a stroll may help you clear your head.

Be aware of your limits. Keep in mind that there are just such a variety of hours in a day. Don't hesitate to state "no" when individuals request that you interpretation of assignments you don't have sufficient energy or vitality to finish.

Keep a diary. Composing sometimes helps people organize their contemplations and think of down to earth arrangements. Expounding on your musings, emotions and recollections can likewise fortify your soul.

Open up to loved ones. Ask friends or relatives on the off chance that they would be "accessible if the need arises" in times of stress. Then again arrange a standard "registration" time when you can get together or call each other.

A few Emotions the Caregiver May Experience

At the point when caring for a friend or family member with cancer, caregivers may feel:

Guilt: Sometimes parental figures feel regretful that they are sound. Others may feel severe about appreciating things in life that their adored one can't. It is additionally basic for guardians to feel that they are not doing what's needed to offer assistance.

Anger: Caregivers may feel angry with cancer itself, or with themselves, their cherished one, relatives, specialists or others. Pinpointing the wellspring of the outrage can help you better deal with the inclination.

Sadness: It's common to feel tragic when somebody you adore is genuinely sick. You may likewise miss the life you two had before cancer.

Stress/ Worry: now and again, you may feel tense, anxious or terrified or experience issues unwinding. This is typical. Cases of things guardians frequently stress over incorporate their loved one's wellbeing, paying the bills and how other relatives are coping.

Debilitation: Being a caregiver can here and there feel like a long, uneven street. It's anything but difficult to get disheartened every now and then. This is particularly valid if your cherished one's condition turns more terrible.

Feeling overwhelmed: It is normal to feel overwhelmed as a guardian. Giving pragmatic and enthusiastic support to somebody with tumor can feel like an all day work.

Could It Be Depression?

It is typical to feel tragic or irate when a friend or family member has the tumor. In any case, converse with your specialist in the event that you have any of these emotions or side effects for over two weeks:

Feeling overpowered or powerless

Prolonged times of crying

Inability to appreciate things

Difficulty concentrating

Trouble dozing or resting excessively

Upset stomach

Weight misfortune or weight pick up

Thoughts of harming yourself

These might be indications of depression, and help is accessible, converse with your specialist to locate the best treatment for you.

Consider building up your spiritual side: For a few people, this implies partaking in religious exercises. Others discover the deep sense of being in workmanship or nature. Regardless of what your convictions are, building up your otherworldly side could give comfort during this time.

Converse with a health care professional about your sentiments and stresses: Numerous parental figures feel overpowered and alone. You may require more than companions or relatives to converse with. Talking with a guide or oncology social laborer may help you adapt to some of your sentiments and stresses. Disease Care's oncology social specialists are only a phone call away.

Join a care group for caregivers: Chatting with different caregivers can likewise help you feel less alone. Cancer Care offers free up close and personal, phone and online care groups for parental figures. These gatherings give a place of refuge where you can share your worries and gain from other people who are experiencing comparable circumstances.

Go easy on yourself: Once in a while, you may feel you could have accomplished something in an unexpected way. Make an effort not to be too hard on yourself. Concentrate on all the positive things you are accomplishing for your loved one.

Getting Help with Care giving Responsibilities

As a caregiver figure, it is vital to know and acknowledge your own points of confinement. Having an emotionally supportive network is a piece of dealing with your loved one and yourself. Choose which errands you will do all alone and which you will require help with.

Here are a few things you can do that will help you in your part as a caregiver:

Check with family and companions. Are there any relatives, companions, individuals from your confidence group, associates? Regularly individuals need to offer assistance. You simply need to inquire. Be particular about the sort of help you need, and keep records of who is taking care of what task.

Find out about break mind programs. Reprieve care gives family and companions a reprieve from care giving. While you run errands or take some individual time, rest parental figures invest energy with your adored one briefly. They may help with encouraging, showering or everyday schedules. Request a referral from a human services proficient, companion or nearby administration organization.

Know your rights. On the off chance that you work for an organization with at least 50 representatives and have worked there for no less than one year, you are most likely permitted unpaid leave under the Family and Medical Leave Act to give care to your loved one. Many smaller companies permit their workers to utilize sick days and vacations for care giving purposes. Approach your human resources division for encouraging and to see if this law applies to your organization.

CHAPTER 7. 7 KEY RISK FACTORS FOR CANCERS YOU MUST KNOW

Many erroneously hold the view that each swelling or bump is cancer. In any case, this is not so. Unlike benign swellings, dangerous cells, for the most part, tend to attack encompassing tissues and at times metastasize to remove body tissues through the circulation system or lymphatic framework. Cancers result when there is a disturbance to the typical procedure of cell division. Body cells are consistently experiencing cell division, but in a controlled way to supplant maturing and dead cells. Nonetheless, a blame or change now and again happens amid this procedure, if not quickly repaired by the body, this outcome in the development of unusual cells which keep on proliferating wildly and eventually prompt to Cancers.

Accordingly, the health weight of cancer is enormous. Cancer is said to kill a greater number of individuals every year than HIV/AIDS, Malaria, and Tuberculosis. As indicated by the International Agency for Research on Cancer (IARC), by 2030, more than 21 million new instances of the tumor would have been determined to have 13 million individuals biting the dust from malignancy consistently.

A perplexing interchange of several risk factors, some of which are talked about underneath figures out who contracts disease and who does not:

Smoking

Cigarette smoking, dynamic or uninvolved is embroiled in many tumors including lung, nasopharyngeal, oesophageal and prostate malignancies to say a couple. Truth be told, explore has demonstrated that around 33% of all yearly tumor passings in the United States come about because of smoking. Roughly 98% of patients with Small Cell Lung Cancer (SCLC) have a noteworthy smoking history and luckily, suspension of smoking has corresponded with enhanced survival in these patients.

Obesity

Contrasted and individuals of typical weight and Body Mass Index (BMI), fat people stand a more serious danger of some cancer types including cancers of the pancreas, colon, kidneys, throat, bosom and the endometrium among others. One clarification that has been proposed for this expanded hazard is that fat tissues deliver over the top amounts of estrogen in large individuals. High estrogen levels have been connected with expanded danger of bosom and endometrial growths. Moreover, fat people will probably have raised blood levels of insulin and Insulin-like Growth Factor 1 (IGF-1) which support the advancement of a few malignancies. Considers have demonstrated that overweight and fat people stand 200-400% higher danger of endometrial disease than their partners with a typical BMI.

HIV/AIDS

Immunodeficient people, for example, individuals living with HIV/AIDS are at more danger of building up specific sorts of the tumor. Three of these growths, in particular, Kaposi Sarcoma, Non-Hodgkin Lymphoma and Cervical Cancer are alluded to as AIDS-characterizing ailments. For example, an individual tainted with HIV has a few thousands higher danger of showing Kaposi Sarcoma and 70 times higher danger of creating Non-Hodgkin Lymphoma. Some other tumor sorts they are at danger of incorporate butt-centric cancer, Hodgkin lymphoma, and lung cancer. Since HIV/AIDS debilitates the resistant framework, it is trusted that it inclines to some different contaminations that can bring about cancer e.g. Human Papilloma Virus (HPV) disease that has been ensnared in cervical cancer.

Excessive Alcohol Intake

Studies have demonstrated that extreme utilization of liquor builds your danger of oral, throat, oesophageal and liver cancer. Thus, on the off chance that you quit overabundance drinking, your danger of these deadly cancers will be fundamentally less.

Excessive exposure to Sunlight

People that open themselves to exceptional daylight inadvertently increase their danger of skin cancers. Various reviews have embroiled Ultraviolet (UV) radiation in the pathology of skin cancers, including melanoma. Melanin is a characteristic skin color that offers critical assurance from bright beams. This is the reason light-cleaned individuals who have less melanin color in their skin will probably encounter sunburn and skin cancer.

Positive Family History

For most cancers, people who have at least one close relative (particularly first-degree relatives) that have been determined to have such cancers have a fundamentally higher hazard. Such individuals are said to be hereditarily inclined in light of the fact that they may have acquired a portion of the irregular qualities. For example, a family history of breast cancer in a first-degree relative is one of the essential hazard components for this cancer. On the off chance that a mother or sister is influenced by bosom cancer, the lifetime danger of building up the sickness is expanded by four folds.

Increasing Age

As people increase in age, their danger of growing most cancers likewise tends to increase. For instance, while breast cancer is extremely uncommon in ladies below 25 years, the rate achieves a level in ladies matured 50-55 years. Moreover, prostate cancer is an ailment condition that is normally found in the elderly (Age >65 years) and the pervasiveness can be as high as 80% at 80 years old.

CHAPTER 8. THE CANCER SIGNS

Cancer is one of the leading causes of death in humans. Some might not be able to notice it at first and would likely treat it as a simple illness but little do they know it has become one of the deadliest diseases known to man. It is of utmost importance that you know the signs and symptoms of cancer and what you can do if you discover such signs and symptoms.

Everyone who has cancer will lose some weight at some point in their lives but when you lose weight of about 10 pounds without any apparent reason less than one month is a true sign of cancer. Most often it is a sign of liver and pancreatic cancer.

Another common sign of cancer is when you have a low-grade fever for a span of time from the first you develop the fever up until the next sign of cancer. Fever makes it hard for the body to fight off infection and fever might be a sign of leukemia or lymphoma.

Sudden fatigue or extreme tiredness can become a sign of cancer. If you find it hard to get better from fatigue even with hours of rest, then it might be a sign of cancer. Some colon cancer and blood cancer can be the result of this sign and symptom.

Pain is another common sign of cancer. When you have chronic pain like a headache that does not go away with simple treatment can become a sign and symptom of cancer. Back pain can be a symptom of cancer in the colon or in the ovary.

When you find a sore that does not seem to heal, you should try to check it out with your doctor. A long-lasting sore in the mouth can be a sign of oral cancer from people who smoke or chew nicotine gums. Sores found in the vaginal area can become cancer or signs of infection. Have yourself checked by the doctor?

If you find yourself having unusual bleeding or discharges during urination, you might want to consult your doctor. If you have bloody discharges when you cough, it might be a sign of lung cancer and if you have blood in your stool, it can be colon cancer.

Learning the common signs and symptoms of cancer is crucial as cancer can be managed and even destroyed when they are discovered at the early stage. Be more sensitive to your body and if you discover the signs and symptoms above, talk to your doctor.

Seven Signs of Cancer in Women

There are a few types of cancer that are regularly found in ladies, which incorporate bosom, cervical, ovarian, vaginal, and colon growth. As a lady, you have to know the notice indications of each of those maladies to have the capacity to keep them from happening. In the event that you encounter any of these indications and you speculate that you may have cancer, you ought to see a specialist quickly. Chances are, you might not have it, but rather it's ideal to be protected than too bad.

Here are seven indications of disease in women you ought to know:

1. Pelvic Pain

Women normally feel pelvic agony (torment or weight beneath the navel) before or amid their month to month time frame. Be that as it may, if the torment holds on even after you've had your period; it could be an indication of endometrial, ovarian, cervical, fallopian tube, or vaginal cancer.

2. Stomach Swelling and Bloating

This is a typical indication of ovarian cancer. Some of the time it is trailed by a determined lower back agony too. Despite the fact that bloating is ordinarily connected to acid reflux, you can't simply disregard it. Particularly in the event that it gets so awful that you can't catch your pants.

3. Strange Vaginal Bleeding

This could be a symptom of gynecologic cancer, particularly when you have a substantial periods and seeping between periods. Bleeding amid and after sex could likewise show and connection to cervical, uterine, and ovarian cancer.

4. Constant Fever

You ought to counsel a specialist in the event that you have had fever for over 7 days. It may be an indication of cancer, yet it could likewise be brought about by different less life-debilitating ailment. A steady stomach upset or gut change amid the fever is something you ought to likewise stress about. Constipation, the runs, tooting, or ridiculous stool could be an indication of colon cancer.

5. Unintentional Weight Loss

In the event that you lose at least 10 pounds without attempting (no work out, no eating routine), you ought to see a specialist to counsel about the likelihood of having cancer. Besides, genuine weight reduction could likewise demonstrate the phase of the cancer.

6. Variations from the norm in the Vulva or Vagina

Vulva or vaginal variations from the norm could be a manifestation of vaginal cancer. These could be as bruises, rankle, changes in skin shading, and strange release. Standard registration with a gynecologist can help you avoid gynecologic cancer.

7. Changes in the Breast

Women are encouraged to perform consistent bosom self-examination. You ought to search for any knots, soreness, dimpling, swelling or areola release. On the off chance that you watch any adjustments in your bosom, you ought to report it to a specialist quickly.

Is Back Pain A Sign Of Cancer?

The majority of back pain cases in the U.S. are named idiopathic, which means no correct reason for agony is found. Those with waiting, unexplained back agony may create fears that the cause is something genuine like cancer.

Back pain is one conceivable manifestation of types of cancer, however this is genuinely uncommon. A recent report entitled " Cancer as a reason for back agony: recurrence, clinical presentation, and demonstrative systems" observed growth to be the reason for back torment in 13 out of 1,975 patients (.66%). In spite of the fact that uncommon, it is vital to comprehend when and how back agony might be symptomatic of various types of cancer, both to facilitate your mind when it is not and to encourage early location when it is.

Back pain can emerge from malignancy in two fundamental ways:

Pain might be from tumors in close-by organs that press on muscles and nerves of the back and

Pain can emerge from tumors in the spine itself.

Referred Pain

Tumors are anomalous tissue developments. At the point when tumors develop on the colon, rectum, ovary, pancreas or kidney, agony might be felt in the hips; bring down back and additionally mid back. Tumors on the lungs can bring about torment in the upper back.

On the off chance that torment is connected with tumors in close-by organs, it won't be the main manifestation you have. Growth side effects shift contingent upon the kind of malignancy bringing on them. A few manifestations that are shared by many types of cancer are:

Unexplained weight reduction

Fever

Weariness

Chills

Skin changes (blushing, obscuring, yellowing, or over the top hair development)

Nausea

Vomiting

Changes in bowel function that last past a month or blood in the stool may demonstrate colon disease. Blood in the pee or changes in passing pee can demonstrate bladder or prostate cancer. Strange vaginal release may show tumor of the cervix. Drawn out pelvic agony may demonstrate growth of the uterus or ovaries. Hacking up blood is a side effect of lung cancer.

Remember that each of these side effects might be brought on by an option that is other than cancer. Whatever the cause, a trek to the specialist is all together. The sooner the cause is found, the faster you can seek after effective treatment.

Spinal Tumors

Tumors on the spine might be dangerous (carcinogenic) or kind (non-harmful). Harmful tumors on the spine are most normally the aftereffect of metastasis (spreading) of growth from another part of the body, yet may likewise come about because of cancer of the spine itself.

The three types of spinal tumors are vertebral section tumors, intradural-extramedullary tumors, and intramedullary tumors. Vertebral segment tumors grow either on the vertebra or the spinal circle. Intradural-extramedullary tumors become further inside the spine but outside the spinal cord (nerves). Intramedullary tumors occur directly close by spinal nerves and are most regular in the neck.

Torment from spinal tumors does not decrease with rest and might be more awful at morning and night. Tumors can bring about nerve pressure and prompt to torment, shortcoming or deadness that goes along the influenced nerve's pathway. There is by and large serious torment at the site of the tumor when weight is connected. Bowing and curving might be particularly excruciating. These indications are dependably a reason for concern whether connected with tumors or not, and analysis ought to be looked for. These manifestations are well on the way to be connected with cancer on the off chance that they happen with other common cancer symptoms.

CHAPTER 9. FIVE ALL-STAR FOODS TO HELP PREVENT CANCER

Cancer is a standout amongst the most widely recognized incessant maladies in the United States and its predominance is developing. It's assessed that 1 in 2 men and ladies will be determined to have growth amid their lifetime, and in 2010 alone more than 1.5 million new cases were diagnosed.

With numbers like these, you may feel cancer is only an unavoidable truth and you're generally defenseless to impact your hazard. While there are surely hazard elements you can't control, similar to family history or ethnic foundation, you ought to realize that there are similarly the same number of - if not more - that you can... furthermore, a standout amongst the most powerful is your eating diet.

"Scientific evidence recommends that around 33% of the 569,490 cancer deaths anticipated that would happen in 2010 will be identified with overweight or heftiness, physical inertia, and poor sustenance and along these lines could likewise be counteracted."

For all fruits and veggies are awesome decisions for a cancer preventive eating routine; however there are sure foods that are veritable all-stars with regards to keeping malignancy away. On the off chance that you need to give your family's eating routine some additional disease-battling punch, attempt to consolidate a portion of the accompanying elite player foods into your meals.

Tomatoes

Tomatoes are a rich source of lycopene, an antioxidant carotenoid that gives them their red color. Lycopene is a powerhouse antioxidant that has been found to protect cells and DNA from damage, while also suppressing tumor growth. One of the reasons for the abnormal growth of cells, which can lead to cancerous tumors, is poor communication between cells; it's thought that lycopene may stimulate cell-to-cell communication and thereby suppress tumor growth.

Both animal and human studies have found lycopene from tomatoes may help prevent colorectal, prostate, breast, endometrial, lung, cervical, stomach and pancreatic cancers.

A few tips: Cooked tomatoes, such as those in pasta sauce, tomato juice, ketchup, etc., contain higher concentrations of lycopene than raw tomatoes, so you may get more of this beneficial compound by eating your tomatoes cooked. You'll also want to eat your tomatoes with some olive oil or other fat, as lycopene is a fat-soluble nutrient that requires fat in order to be properly absorbed by your body.

Raspberries

Raspberries are an excellent source of ellagic acid, a phytochemical that has shown potent anti-cancer effects. To date, research has shown ellagic acid may help fight cancer by:

Acting as an antioxidant

Causing cell death to cancer cells

Reducing the effect of estrogen in promoting growth of breast cancer cells

Helping your liver to break down and remove cancer-causing substances from your body

Inhibiting the growth of tumors

Along with raspberries, ellagic acid can also be found in strawberries, cranberries, walnuts, pecans and pomegranates.

Broccoli Sprouts

You may have heard that cruciferous vegetables like broccoli are great for helping to fight cancer. This is true, but you can take it one step further by eating broccoli in its immature, or sprout, form.

Broccoli sprouts contain glucoraphanin, a precursor to sulforaphane -- a compound known to help your body eliminate cancer-causing compounds and fight free radicals, which can damage DNA, kill cells and potentially lead to cancer.

Sprouts are a particularly concentrated source of nutrients and gram for gram they contain more potentially cancer-fighting compounds than mature broccoli. One study even found that eating slightly more than 100 grams of broccoli, radish, alfalfa and clover sprouts a day for 14 days was enough to provide a protective effect.

If you're new to sprouts, try adding them to salads and sandwiches for a tasty and ultra-healthy treat.

Cruciferous Veggies

As mentioned above, cruciferous vegetables like broccoli, cauliflower, Brussels sprouts, kale, cabbage, and bok choy are also widely known for their cancer-fighting capabilities. Studies have linked the consumption of cruciferous veggies with a reduced risk of colon, lung, bladder, breast, prostate, and other cancers.

The beneficial effects come, in part, from indole-3-carbinol and isothiocyanates. These glucosinolates are formed when the vegetables are chopped or chewed, and studies show they offer a protective effect against cancer.

Indole-3-carbinol may help deactivate an estrogen metabolite that promotes tumor growth, especially in breast cells, while increasing the level of a form of estrogen that may protect against cancer. This compound may also help stop the movement of cancer cells to other parts of your body.

Further, a study funded by the National Cancer Institute found that eating 1 to 2 cups of cruciferous vegetables a day resulted in a 22 percent drop in oxidative stress, which has been linked to a range of diseases including cancer, diabetes, Alzheimer's disease and rheumatoid arthritis.

Garlic

The sulfur-containing compounds that give garlic its pungent odor are also responsible for its role as a cancer-fighting food. The National Cancer Institute "recognizes garlic as one of the several vegetables with potential anticancer properties," noting that garlic may help support good health by:

Blocking the formation of cancer-causing substances

Halting the activation of cancer-causing substances

Enhancing DNA repair

Reducing cell proliferation

Inducing cell death

Providing antibacterial properties

Population studies have shown that increased intake of garlic may help reduce the risk of several types of cancer, including stomach, colon, esophagus, pancreas, and breast.

THE END

Printed in Great Britain
by Amazon